Osteoarthritis – (Arthrose in Europe)

How to prevent and treat this disease accordingly

Constantin Panow, MD

COPYRIGHT 2018

"Strength which is in every one of us is our only healer."

Hippocrates (460-370BC)

Copyright 2018

Disclaimer

Archeology

Geography

First

Nutriments

Description

Immunity

Evolution

Medicine

Future developments

History

Prevalence

Gout

Fish

Motivation

Inflammation issue

Cardio-vascular

Teeth hygiene

Starches

Nutritional proposal

Fasting

Type of lipids

Fruit

Infection

Cardiac infarction

Cartilage

Ligaments

Sports

Metabolism

Faulty joint adaptation

Economy

Age

Youngsters

Radiology

Rare disease

Other

Uncommon syndromes

Fine characteristics

Additional incentives

Website

DISCLAIMER

Author and publisher decline responsibility about any wrong understanding or interpretation and consequent faulty application of rules of following text.

This booklet is for information purposes only.

ARCHEOLOGY

Osteoarthritis has always been a common disease, but archeology does not supply many examples of it.

Obviously, this disease was less frequent in Antiquity.

GEOGRAPHY

Distribution over the Globe is also uneven, owing to the fact of different ways of living.

FIRST

Most important factor is probably Nutrition.

NUTRIMENTS

Tightly linked to high protein diets, especially meat, nowadays' human, in industrialized countries, is heavily burdened by Pseudo- gout.

Also called Chondro-calcinosis, this illness characterizes itself by deposition of Pyrophosphate crystals in articulations.

DESCRIPTION

Manifesting as bouts of inflammation in joints, with effusion followed by slow improvement, flare-up responds well to anti-inflammatory drugs (AINS).

IMMUNITY

Specifically, this paradigm of osteoarthritis is typically a model of an autoimmune ailment.

Most important factor is heavy red meat consumption.

Poultry is a bit better in this respect, but not a lot.

Dairy products can also trigger accesses of sickness.

Fish can be consumed in much higher proportions without adverse effects.

Protein source from Invertebrates is probably a better solution.

Snails, mussels, Clams, calamari, octopus, crabs are probably much healthier.

EVOLUTION

If we analyze those facts, we observe, that farther we humans are from viewpoint of evolution from species, which gives origin to nutriment, safer this product is.

Or, to put it as a patient of mine said: "In fact we practice a low-grade cannibalism".

MEDICINE

As for instance, a porcine heart valve can stay in our bodies for decades without being deformed by autoimmune process, as it is considered as "self" by our immune system.

Today, diabetics use genetically produced human insulin, but for decades this group of patients was using porcine, or even bovine hormone without knowledgeable side-effects.

FUTURE DEVELOPMENTS

Genetically, we are different from other mammals by only a small percentage of DNA, and present many similarities, inviting modern scientists to think that one day organ transplants from other species wouldn't be pure speculation.

HISTORY

Until recent centuries, peasants in Europe would make a feast of red meat only once or twice per year.

At beginning of twentieth century people would consume a lot of fruit and vegetables, which was responsible, for instance, for urinary bladder stones. (Oxalate).

Something I haven't observed even once in my career of almost 40 years.

PREVALENCE

Pseudo-gout can be recorded in more than 70% of patients above 70.

-And osteoarthritis in over 60% after 60 years of age.

GOUT

In fact, Pseudo-gout is a misnomer, as it is very common, unlike gout, which is rare.

But common nutrition lines remain.

FISH

Here is to be said that fish and its oil have an anti-inflammatory effect on their own, counteracting the link with proteins.

MOTIVATION

One of main reasons why I decided to write this short text, is that I hear about colleagues, who even in nowadays advanced scientific world say to their patient they have nothing to propose as therapy.

Of course, if you consider osteoarthritis spurs are almost not absorbable, not so with inflammatory bouts and their prevention.

Ok, treatment with drugs stops the spurt, but leaves a low-grade disease effect.

INFLAMMATION ISSUE

Modern laboratories are even able to show this irritation of tissues.

CARDIO-VASCULAR

Recent research points that not only inflammation is not irrelevant, but that it is one of main factors, which trigger cardio-vascular disease.

Be it thrombo-embolism or coronary infarcts, stroke, and atherosclerosis, they all depend heavily on this influence.

TEETH HYGIENE

Literature discloses that teeth hygiene is an essential part in this respect.

Porphyromonas gingivalis can promote and exacerbate arterial plaques.

Or, as an elderly lady in my colleague's practice misunderstood, when he told her she had osteoarthritis: "Oh, my Gosh, and my husband died from it!"

As arthrose and atherosclérose (French) sound akin.

As you can observe for yourself, she was not completely wrong.

Teeth granulomas have been a long-known cause of early osteoarthritis.

STARCHES

Second most important aspect of Chondro-calcinosis is that it is tightly associated with starch carbohydrate utilization.

I remember still a few patients who would absorb neither too much meat, nor cheese or poultry, and who would suffer from this disease.

Gluten contained in its highest concentration in wheat is an important trigger.

White bread, pasta and pizzas are thus concerned.

Potatoes are a better solution in moderate amounts. There is a big choice of Gluten-free cereals.

White rice consumption is to be discouraged from, as it possesses an extremely high glycemic index.

Beware also about lectins contained in some food, which have the same inflammatory effect as gluten.

Internet provides precise information about this topic.

Here, again, you see closeness to autoimmune

disease.

I remember, after having discussed this topic for a while with one of my patients, he would ask obviously desperate:

"So, what, for God's sake am I going to eat?"

NUTRITIONAL PROPOSAL

Don't worry!

This issue is easy to solve, and at your best advantage.

There are two types of Carbohydrates, Starch- and Fiber-carbohydrates.

Consider glycemic index, and you would see that second ones are much healthier.

Start by cutting away completely simple sugar from your diet! You can use Stevia as a sweetener, without calories.

Glucose as such is toxic for cartilage.

But you must adapt your body little by little, without being in a hurry, as hypoglycemia can be serious.

Start by halving at first supply in pasta, rice, bread, and potatoes!

Then you can reduce those four progressively to

zero.

Besides, your brain is mostly composed of lipids, and if you increase fat consumption it would be happier.

And you would feel healthier, in better mood.

FASTING

Fasting is also important in this process, especially to lose excessive weight, this being by itself component of joint disease.

While off-food hours, your organism produces so-called ketone bodies, which are nothing else than lipids.

On which your brain learns progressively to thrive.

TYPE OF LIPIDS

Try to adjust accordingly type of lipids you ingest!

- As proportion of saturated, towards mono-unsaturated and poly-unsaturated fats is important.

This thematic could be a book-project on its own.

A good balance of such ones is decisive for articular health.

But beware, as soon you heat unsaturated fat, you destroy Essential Fatty Acids contained.

This is not a simple topic, as there is little literature available, and it is completely unclear what percentage should be dedicated to one or the other.

As a rule, animal fat causes inflammation while sea- food and vegetal oils soothe this one.

FRUIT

Those contain fructose, which is better than glucose, but owing to similarities should probably be limited in quantity.

Apart from that, some fruit is a Lectins source.

Whole fruit is to be preferred to juice.

INFECTION

Another element pertaining to osteoarthritis is that any inflammation of every cause is potential promoter.

Thus, people who eat a lot of under-cooked meat or poultry, harbor for long periods in their bodies *Campylobacter jejuni.*

This is rather an innocuous germ, exceedingly common, and for children with this kind of gastro-enteritis it is not mandatory to deliver antibiotics.

But on the long run, you can see big spurs emerging from vertebral bodies, called spondylophytes.

Another interesting microbe is *Mycoplasma pneumoniae.*

It is a bug between virus and bacterium, rather second but with obligatory intra-cellular replication.

Surface cellular resemblance to male genitals makes it ubiquitous and more prevalent in men than in women.

Hence, your grandfather's "low grade" almost constant cough, especially during the bad season.

Here again, articular pain at the same time, most frequently in lower back, is almost pathognomonic.

-So-called "facet syndrome". Sputum is sparse and white.

Sometimes, thoracic pain, or tinnitus are present.

A tight link exists with atherosclerotic complications, be it stroke or myocardial infarction.

CARDIAC INFARCTION

Thus, if micro-organisms from teeth are arterial plaque etiology.

Vessel thrombosis is most of the time probably due to cold agglutinins from Mycoplasmas.

As soon as they find to anchor on arterial wall, blood flow becomes sluggish, and vessel lumen closes.

This is the case especially at night when body temperature goes down with deep sleep.

Statistical relationship of cardio-vascular events and cold season has been known for a long time.

CARTILAGE

If simple sugars and starch are deleterious for your joints.

Fresh salad and vegetables cooked or raw are essential for their health.

Cartilage is much better protected and becomes more resilient and tough in texture with their consumption.

Many vegetables contain a high amount of natural Mucopolysaccharides, as for instance Okra (Bamja) and Courgette (Zucchini).

Those ones, as vegetables in general, are beneficial to articulations.

Leaves of the Linden tree are also especially rich in this component.

Apart from drinking it as tea, we eat its leaves in spring, in a similar way as rolled vine leaves (Sarmi).

Articular fluid, which nourishes cartilage, contains similar components produced by human body.

Hence, the best advice I can give you, to prevent, or even treat Osteoarthritis, is increasing greens (salad), vegetables and raw vegetal oils consumption.

Beware of urinary oxalate stones on a vegetarian diet!

Absorb enough liquid! A soup with main meals is an excellent habit.

Drinking three liters per day is probably a good measure, but you must consider expenditure.

LIGAMENTS

Loosening of articular capsules and ligaments is another feature of pseudo-gout, which contributes to osteophyte formation.

SPORTS

As to physical activity, this is second most important element for evolution of disease.

With incremental progression of loading, sportsmen and –women do not have adverse effects of excessive protein consumption.

Though, this is still a topic of debate, medical practitioners observe many cases of chondro-calcinosis among athletes.

Especially those involved in aerobic exercise are commonly concerned.

Thus, with many other medical workers and trainers, I would rather recommend anaerobic activity for prevention and disease treatment.

I.E. strength training.

Intense and short sets entailing several body parts, is what is proposed most.

Walking, on the other hand has a stabilizing joint effect, and should not be neglected.

It also is presumed to be a cartilage strengthening

method.

CONSTANTIN PANOW

METABOLISM

From another point of view, Pseudo-gout is typically a metabolic ailment.

It is tightly linked to diabetes, arterial hypertension, and high cholesterol in blood.

Thus, also obesity plays a non-negligible role.

FAULTY JOINT ADAPTATION

A different eliciting factor of osteoarthritis is articular adaptation of bone.

Imperfections on this level are heavily paid for with cartilage and bone erosion.

This being especially true for scoliosis in its excessive forms.

ECONOMY

Unnecessary to say, how high economical costs of these disturbances are.

From simple consultation in general practitioners' office, the spectrum finishes in the operating room for hip prosthesis, for instance.

AGE

Despite it is the prerogative of elderly people, chondro- calcinosis can concern all age groups.

If younger patients are involved with this disease, medical doctors should search for hemosiderosis (iron overload) or Wilson's disease (copper metabolism disturbance).

YOUNGSTERS

This is especially true in patients before 30 years of lifetime.

Thus, you see how important precision of diagnosis is!

RADIOLOGY

Fine cartilage calcifications can be observed with radiography, scanner and ultrasound.

But more importantly is diagnosis of facet syndrome, and especially *facet-osteoarthritis*.

This last one is most frequent consequence of pseudo-gout.

When it is perceived in the cervical spine in a patient before 30 years of age, diagnosis of this entity is almost certain.

RARE DISEASE

More frequently due to hemosiderosis, than Wilson's disease, it readily responds to bloodletting.

Other

Of course, any inflammation of articulations, as rheumatoid arthritis, for instance, ends up in osteoarthritis.

Another entity is neuropathic disease, which induces joint misalignment first, then partition of bone ends.

This one vaguely resembles osteoarthritis but is no match for the experienced eye of a well-informed radiologist.

UNCOMMON SYNDROMES

Like Ehlers-Danlos and similar, are out of the scope of this short text.

Gout for itself, has specific drug therapies, depending on level of uric acid in blood.

FINE CHARACTERISTICS

Last, but not least, radiographic features of osteoarthritis are cartilage wear off, joint-space narrowing, para-articular spurs, and bone geodes.

Synovial reaction, hyper-vascularity, and articular cysts and pseudo-cysts, like Baker's, are another attribute.

ADDITIONAL INCENTIVE

I already explained you the reason for which I am writing this exposé, but an alternative one is that I am convinced with Hippocrates that:

"If somebody wishes good health, one should ask him/her first, whether he/she is ready to give up conditions which conducted him/her to this disease."

And besides, I believe that almost no ailment is completely irreversible.

As my practice showed me, at least improvement is always possible.

I hope this short text would help you in your everyday life.

WEBSITE

You can reach me at:

www.thenopillshealthprospect.com

If you have any questions or commentaries, do not hesitate, write to me!

I would be happy to discuss your concern.